THE ELMAN TECHNIQUE

The Basis of Rapid Hypnotherapy

Tim Brunson, PhD

Disclaimer

The content of this book is intended solely for the use of clinicians involved with various integrative medical disciplines. This book is not intended for the general public. Clinicians using the content contained herein take sole responsibility for any claims arising from this material.

The International Hypnosis Research Institute, LLC

600 Leighton Avenune, Suite C

Anniston, Alabama 36207

http://www.hypnosisresearchinstitute.org

CONTENTS

INTRODUCTION

Like most of the American public, misconceptions led me to be more than suspicious of the field called hypnosis. Months into a Neuro-Linguistic Programming practitioner course, our instructor Clinton Clay discussed that NLP's origin and development was partially derived from a study of Milton H. Erickson, MD, who is regarded as the Father of American Hypnotherapy. During the class Clay discussed many of the master's linguistic techniques. Later, as I sat in a local Huntsville, Alabama, restaurant having lunch with my fellow students, I asked, "What just happened to us?"

Apparently, while discussing Erickson's methods our instructor had changed our mental state placing us in a mild form of trance. Although I was relieved that I had not lost control of my will or "quacked like a duck", I was intrigued with the nature of hypnosis.

After I finished a subsequent NLP master practitioner course, I was drawn to take a course offered in nearby Atlanta. Sponsored by the American Institute of Hypnotherapy, a young hypnotist named Topher Morrison wowed the class with demonstrations of the power of hypnosis. While his focus was on the techniques of Al Krasner, PhD, AIH's founder, Morrison admitted that his "hero" was a former stage hypnotist by the name of David Elman. This prompted me to immediately purchase a copy of Elman's book, which had been published under the title <u>Hypnotherapy</u>. (The original edition was titled <u>Findings in Hypnosis</u>.)

My studies of hypnosis have continued. Over the next several years I studied Ericksonian hypnosis with Topher Morrison, who was then a Doctor of Clinical Hypnotherapy, and Bill O'Hanlon, LMFT, who was Erickson's gardener during his college years, and others. I also received instruction in advanced hypnotherapy techniques from Richard Nieves, PhD, as well as taking courses from many others, such as Ernest L. Rossi, Erickson's protégé; Carol Ginandes, PhD, of the Harvard Medical School; and Ted Benton, of Massachusetts General Hospital.

Thanks to my involvement with the National Institutes for the Clinical Study of Behavioral Medicine, the Association for Comprehensive Energy Psychology, the Institute for the Study of Subtle Energies and Energy Medicine, the American Academy of Pain Management, the International Medical and Dental Hypnotherapy Association, the National Guild of Hypnotists, the International Hypnosis Federation, and the American Board of Hypnotherapy, I have had the opportunity to study with a virtual who's who in integrative health care.

Nevertheless, despite the plethora of mind/body techniques to which I have been exposed, I have always been fascinated with the speed and effectiveness of the rapid and instant techniques used by stage hypnotists. Like many of the "serious clinicians", I tended to look down upon my brethren who made their living entertaining audiences with the tricks of hypnosis. I felt that they were cheapening our profession. Then I got to know several of them. A few had dual backgrounds in clinical and stage work. Over the years I have come to respect their abilities.

Thanks to Anne Spencer, PhD, the founder of IMDHA, I was able to locate a set of Elman's 27 audio tapes. Over the course of a few years I listened to them, transcribing all the demonstrations from his original courses, which he gave to medical and dental professionals. Then I had the opportunity to spend a day with Gerald Kein, the Orlando hypnotist who as a young teen participated in recording some of Elman's classes. It was through exhaustive study of Elman's book, repetitive listening of the original recordings, and Kein's expert instruction that I began to fully understand the essence of Elman hypnotherapy.

I have recognized that allopathic medicine, despite its promise and accomplishment, has its limitations. The volume of integrative health care research documented by the National Institutes of Health show that allopathic medicine is not the end-all of the healing professions. As modalities such as energy psychology and energy medicine slowly fight for credibility, I simultaneously see a fascination with the power of hypnosis.

Hypnosis, (or if you prefer "hypnotherapy"), and its cousin "guided imagery" are probably the most powerful and least understood healing modalities available. Nevertheless, the "experts" seem to have forced the evolution of their clinical applications into the quite arbitrary boxes of guided visualization and/or Ericksonian hypnosis. Regardless of the depth and power of those theories, I couldn't help but feel that something was missing. They lacked the ability to get rapid results in time-constrained medical and dental situations. So again, I started looking into techniques of the stage hypnotist and eventually found my way back to Elman, who had trained almost 3,000 medical and dental practitioners in the mid-twentieth century.

Over the years I have met many talented and successful practitioners of guided imagery and Ericksonian hypnosis. Clearly, I applaud their accomplishments and contributions. Many of them are extremely gifted and talented. Others, many of whom possess respected mental health or medical or dental licenses, have delved into hypnosis with only minimal training. I'm surprised that some of them even consider themselves as hypnotherapists. I am happy to say that even these laymen and women are still contributing as healers even with their limited hypnosis knowledge.

My contention is that a truly professional hypnotherapist must be trained in a wide range of topics. This should include medical, neurological, and psychological subjects as well as guided imagery and direct and indirect hypnotic techniques. This should include both an expertise in the techniques and an extensive knowledge of their applications.

For those who are already licensed in the healing modalities and who have no desire to complete the comprehensive training of a clinical hypnotherapist, whether they have had any hypnosis training, the rapid techniques included in Elman hypnotherapy can and will become a valuable addition to their skill set.

I have designed the <u>Elman Hypnotherapy: Beyond the Basics</u> course and written this book for two reasons. First, I want to provide a comprehensive and effective model for training the existing hypnotherapist in these skills. Second, I want to provide a skill-building methodology and manual to help other clinicians broaden their existing knowledge and talents with these wonderful protocols. My hope this that by learning Elman's methodologies, the student and reader can enhance their abilities to heal.

In this series I will present and explain the full range of Elman Hypnotherapy. Though at times I may introduce one of my own theories, I will make every effort to retain the original concepts and techniques the way the master intended.

WHO WAS DAVE ELMAN?

As we begin our study of Elman hypnotherapy, let's start by discussing just who Dave Elman was. He was born in Park River, North Dakota, in 1900. His father was accomplished in the field of hypnosis, which stimulated Elman's interest in the subject early in his life. By the age of eight and a half he had gained the utmost respect for the vast possibilities of hypnosis. His father later became ill and was dying from cancer. A family friend, who was skilled as a stage hypnotist, was able to relieve his father's pain. Young Elman was particularly impressed that his father's pain was relieved by hypnosis rather than traditional medical treatment. It was this that led to his life-long interest in the study of hypnosis.

Elman spent much of his career working as a musician, song writer, and as a radio personality, although he had worked as a stage hypnotist at an early age. In 1948, a group of New Jersey physicians repeatedly approached Elman to encourage him to teach them how to apply hypnosis to the practice of medicine. Though some of them had received training in this area, they were dissatisfied with what they had learned. Eventually Elman decided to design a course on hypnosis. Starting with the first group of 20 New Jersey physicians, he eventually trained thousands of medical doctors, including many psychiatrists, and dentists.

He initially received considerable resistance from some physicians who felt that they could only learn from other medical professional. They quickly came to appreciate his competence and authority regarding the subject. However, his credibility within the medical and dental professions should come as no surprise. Even as a child he studied the works of such medical and psychological professionals as Henry Munro, Bernheim, Liebeult, and others.

WHY STUDY ELMAN TECHNIQUES?

The techniques taught by Dr. Milton Erickson *seem* to be the most popular among many psychologists and medical doctors. Indeed, Ericksonian hypnosis tends to dominate the field of therapeutic and research applications today. Most people do not know that Erickson and Elman were bitter rivals who openly criticized each other's competence and abilities. Theirs was a battle between the psychiatrist and the layman. After hypnosis for medical and psychological treatment was approved by the American Medical Association in 1958 and the American Psychological Association in 1959, interest in Elman waned and Erickson's followers began to dominate the world of hypnotherapy. Erickson's influence grew, and Elman's memory became relegated to a historical footnote until the 1970's when Gerald Kein, a hypnotherapist teaching in Orlando at the time, revived interest in this forgotten master. Since then hypnotherapists around the world have realized that Elman's techniques are unparalleled when speed or depth is essential.

While in many cases the genius of Erickson's methods has proven superior for psychotherapy and with resistant patients, Elman repeatedly proved that his techniques should be the first choice for medical and dental interventions. This is especially true when acute or chronic pain is present. Guided imagery and Ericksonian hypnosis just do not provide the same quick and lasting relief.

THE ELMAN TECHNIQUE

The heart of Elman Hypnotherapy has been labeled the "Elman technique". Elman's methods have achieved a level of hypnosis that is deep and rapid enough for medical and dental procedures. Initially, clinicians should be able to accomplish this induction within 3 minutes. However, as this may be too long for many situations, my goal is for you to develop your hypnotic operator skills to the point that you can complete the hypnotic process, including therapy, within 1 minute. Now, how is this done?

Currently my only intention is to introduce you to Elman's induction. There are many nuances and concepts that will be discussed later in this book *and* in following books in this series.

The induction process used by Elman has seven distinct steps. In order they are the pre-talk, the suspension of the critical faculty, the achievement of physical relaxation, compounding physical relaxation, mental relaxation, the therapy, and closure. What I am going to present to you now is a brief example of the Elman technique. I will follow the demonstration with a few brief comments regarding these seven steps. In other books of this series, I will more fully explain some of the finer points and describe how to modify these techniques based upon the age of the patient or the purpose of the intervention.

DEMONSTRATION

"I am Doctor Thibidoux, and I will be working with you to help you reduce the discomfort in your shoulder. To do this, I'm going to show you how to relax. In fact, I will show you how to relax so completely that you will have no discomfort in your shoulder at all. So, take a long deep breath. That's right. Now, I'm going to bring my hand down and you are going to close your eyes. Relax you eye muscles to the point where they just won't work. Now, when you are sure they won't work, allow that feeling to go right down to your toes. That's right. And, in a moment we are going to do this again. When we do it a second time, you are going to be able to relax yourself ten times deeper than before. Open your eyes, close your eyes. Allow yourself to become covered in a blanket of relaxation. The third time that we do it, you will be able to double the amount of relaxation that you currently have. Open your eyes. Relax. Now I'm going to lift your hand and drop it. As I raise your hand and drop it, your hand will become as limp as a dish rag. When I drop your hand, your eyes will close, and your relaxation will double. Now open your eyes again, and as you close them, your relaxation will double all the way down to your toes."

"Now I want you to count backwards from 100. By the time you get to 97 you will be so relaxed that there will not be any numbers. Hold on to your physical relaxation. Start with the idea of making your mental relaxation happen. One hundred, now double your physical and mental relaxation and watch the numbers slowly disappearing. 99. Now watch them go. 98. Now they'll be gone. 97. Make them disappear. Now. Are they all gone? Good. Let me tell you some of the advantages of relaxation. When you close your eyes and remember

this state of relaxation, nothing will bother you, nothing will disturb you. In fact, in this state you allow any discomfort in your shoulder to quickly and effortlessly fade away permitting total relaxation to return to your mind and body. Now, open your eyes. How do you feel?"

This was a three-minute Elman induction and therapy. Now, you are probably wondering if this works, why it works, and what is the difference between a three minute and a one-minute Elman induction. While much of this will become clearer in the second book, let me review some of the basic concepts of this induction.

REVIEW

Remember I said that there are seven basic steps. Again, these are the pre-talk, suspending the critical faculty, physical relaxation, compounding the physical relaxation, mental relaxation, therapy, and closure. Let's go through each one of them again.

The *pre-talk* is important for establishing rapport, establishing you as an authority, and reducing or preventing fear. It is also where you create expectation. By this time, you probably understand how important that rapport is to any therapeutic relationship. Also, as I will discuss in more detail later, fear - according to Elman - is the one thing that may prevent someone from either going into a trance or achieving enough depth.

You also probably noticed that I took a mini step when I asked the subject to close her eyes and take a long breath. These actions not only continue the operator-subject relationship, but also have a beneficial effect. Closing the eyes helps the subject to focus inward. And, relaxed breathing helps calm the brain as it encourages the brain stem to create more serotonin (the relaxation neurotransmitter). Of course, Elman never talked about neurotransmitters; this is my personal contribution. Please note that eye closure in and of itself is not necessary nor is asking the subject to take a deep, relaxing breath.

The next step, however, is extremely important. According

to Elman, *suspending the critical faculty* permits suggestive thinking. This is one of the most vital concepts in Elman hypnotherapy. So, what is the critical faculty? Sigmund Freud called this "the watcher who guards your subconscious mind". Modern neurology describes this as a "tyranny of the left brain". In any event, Elman was satisfied to explain critical faculty as the part of the conscious brain that interferes with suggestion. I would like to point out here that eye closure is not the only way to do his. In fact, there are an infinite number of ways to suspend the critical faculty. It can even be done with the subject's eyes wide open!

Physical and *mental relaxation* is essential to getting the subject into the somnambulistic state to which Elman frequently refers. As the critical faculty has been suspended at this point, it is easy to lead the subject into physical relaxation merely by suggestion. Using further suggestions to compound the level of physical relaxation assist the subject to the point where there is no interference among stress and the body and the operator's ability to guide the subject toward their desired goal.

Elman knew that mental relaxation was vital to obtaining a somnambulistic trance. Getting the subject to a point where they cannot see the numbers is one way of doing this. I would like to add a few of my own thoughts here. Mental relaxation calms the part of the brain involved in conflict resolution. The actual name of that brain sector is the anterior cingulate cortex or ACC. When it is calm, more energy is available for the rest of the brain, enabling your stress and fear level to decrease. Once a subject mentally relaxes, they are ready for therapy.

In the example induction, I simply gave suggestions that the discomfort would go away. This is the *therapy* step. Notice that I did not use the word pain. Elman admonished his students to never use that word – substituting the word discomfort for it instead. I will cover more about linguistics in another book in this series. Also, note that I gave the subject a post hypnotic suggestion. I suggested that anytime she closed her eyes, the discomfort would fade.

Finally, there is the *closure*. Notice there is nothing fancy here. Elman merely said, "Open your eyes."

THE TWO ESSENTIAL REQUIREMENTS

Throughout, I've been mentioning the one-minute Elman induction. Now you're probably wondering what you will have to cut to fit this induction into one minute. Let me share with you the essential elements of a hypnotic induction according to Dave Elman: *the suspension of the critical faculty and allowance of selective thinking.* Simply put, Elman said that hypnosis occurs when these two factors exist. As you will learn in this series, hypnosis does not necessarily require trance. Later I will dedicate an entire book to the concept of waking hypnosis. If hypnosis is used in conjunction with trance, then the right level of trance must be obtained. Of course, this assumes that the trance state is tested. However, many of the results of a hypnotic trance may also be obtained in waking hypnosis. I know this may sound confusing. But by the end of this series, you will not only feel comfortable with the material, but you will more clearly understand how it fits together.

HOW TO STUDY HYPNOSIS

I conclude this first book by presenting Elman's advice on how to study hypnosis. Elman both encouraged and admonished his medical and dental students to practice the basic technique as often as possible. This means you should practice the technique a minimum of 20 times per week. Moreover, Elman chided his students never to attempt the advanced applications until they were firmly comfortable with the basic technique. Throughout this series I will continue expanding and refining your skills. So, don't go out and attempt the Elman Technique on a patient with acute pain or who is expecting to give birth any day, until we get to that point. Practice frequently, but don't get ahead of your competency level. There will be plenty of time for you to both increase your skills and to increase your range of applications. After all, this is what this series is all about.

At this point, I suggest that you practice the Elman Technique a minimum of three times with different subjects prior to continuing to the next chapter. By doing so, you will gain much better insight into the concepts discussed.

RESOURCES

General

The International Hypnosis Research Institute

IHRI membership

Advanced-Neuro-Noetic-Hypnosis

IHRI Courses

Books, E-books, and Audiobooks:

Sets

Elman Hypnotherapy: Beyond The Basics

The Elman Technique

Hypnosis Concepts

Covert Hypnotherapy

Hypnosis Compounding

Hypnotic Coma

Rapid Hypnosis Techniques

Practical Elman Hypnotherapy

Elman Hypnotherapy: Beyond the Basics (Bundled)

Embracing Ambiguity: The Worlds Of Ericksonian Hypnosis

Dr. Erickson and His Innovative Style of Hypnotherapy

Pattern Interventions in Hypnotherapy

Differences and Sameness in Hypnotherapy

Stories, Metaphors and the Unconscious Mind

The Power of Implications, Ambiguity, and Reframing in Hypnotherapy

Linguistic Techniques in Hypnotherapy

The Phases of Erickson's Therapy

The Elements of Erickson's Trance Induction

Enhancing Performance: Unleashing Your True Potential

Innovations In Mind/Body Therapies

The Neurology of Mind/Body Health

Transformation Revisited

The Immune System Primer

Using Imagery to Heal

A Quick Pain Management Primer

Healing the Body Basics

The Mind, Surgery, and Recovery

Calming Your Gut

Innovations in Mind/Body Therapies (Bundled)

The Neurology Of Suggestion Series

The Neurology of Suggestion

Advanced Hypnotherapy Protocols and Applications

The Neurology of Suggestion Series (Bundled)

The Neurology Of Suggestion Basics

Change: A New Paradigm for Transformation

Brain Potential: Enhancing and Inhibiting for Peak Performance

Reshaping: Changing your Brain and Body

Mastering Change: 10 Principles for Transformation

Achieving Lasting Change: A System for Transformation

Neurology of Suggestion Applications

The Neurology of Suggestion Basics (Bundled)

Neuro Linguistic Programming Basics

Mastering the NLP Communication Model

Developing Instant Rapport

The Basis of NLP Techniques

Modeling Behavior

Practical NLP Applications

Neuro Linguistic Programming Basics (Bundled)

Individual Books

Advanced Hypnotherapy Script Writing Techniques

Clinical Hypnotherapy Fundamentals

Healing the Body

Healing the Mind

New Directions in Hypnotherapy

Rapid Change: The Secrets of Lasting Personal and Group Transformation

Space/Time-based Interventions: Simple techniques that enhance hypnotherapy